The EDS and Hypermobility ~~~~~~~ ~~~~

By
Lynne D M Noble

Copyright 2018 Lynne D M Noble

This book shall not, by way of trade or otherwise, be lent, re-sold, hired out, or otherwise circulated without the prior consent of the copyright holder or the publisher in any form of binding or cover than that in which it is published and without a similar condition including this condition being imposed on the subsequent purchaser.
 The use of its contents in another medium is also subject to the same conditions.

Independently published

Dedication

To Jude who inspired me to write this book

Acknowledgement

There are probably far too many people who need acknowledging for inspiring me to write this book. I first had the idea to write this book when I had come across one too many people who had EDS or Hypermobility Syndrome and all said that they had been informed that there was no treatment for it and they lived in what amounted to a 'constant sea of pain'.

The composition of connective tissue is not complex by any means but when we look at our current diets it is easy to see how these disorders can manifest themselves since 'progress' has taken many of these essential building blocks out of our diet. Further, we learn little about nutrition nowadays. We were better equipped during the years of the second World War, when obtaining correct nutrition was of paramount importance in times of limited food availability.

We collected rose hips for vitamin C and were given a daily dose of vitamin D in the form of cod liver oil. Yes, we knew about nutrition alright!

Now we need to learn about it again to build up healthy connective tissue and guts. I must acknowledge Jude, a childhood friend, and Carol D, a distant cousin, for giving me the impetus to write this book.

Preface

There is no doubt that thousands of working hours are lost every year due to chronic or acute pain of the joints and surrounding tissues, fatigue, gastrointestinal problems among others which are associated with the hypermobility syndromes.

Once thought to be the result of defective genes – which just had to be 'lived with' there is now increasing recognition that nutritional deficiencies play a part in the symptoms displayed in these syndromes. As such, a change in diet may mean that many of the problems associated with hypermobility syndromes can be attenuated, or disappear altogether, once normal tissue composition has been restored.

Our diets have changed a great deal in the last fifty years. Many of the foods which we ate in the immediate post war years have now been relegated to the diets of the poor or are now the domain of the very elderly who were brought up on food that the current generation are unlikely to eat.

Indeed, many of these foods, which would promote good tissue development, are unobtainable in the supermarket nowadays and I do not know of anyone who makes bone broth which is one of those essentials if you have a connective tissue disorder. Bone broth was the stalwart mainstay of every self- respecting housewife in the war and immediate post war period. Now this 'medicine' is thrown away - for that is indeed what bone broth is - it is medicine for those with poorly developed connective tissue. However, this isn't its only use. There would be less osteoarthritis if we returned to our way of using every available part of an animal in our diet.

Today, I tried to buy fish heads to make fish head soup – another dish full of gelatin – and was thwarted. Long gone are the days when housewives would have a couple of fish heads wrapped up in greaseproof just ready to turn into a warming and healthy soup. I think these skills are now the domain of the very elderly or the professional cooks that you see on the television. We need to learn these skills once again. They need to be taught in schools as a major part of the curriculum. We need to learn what *healthy eating* really is, once again.

The current way of eating effectively removes three of the four main substances required for making healthy connective tissue from the diet. This means that our current 'healthy' diets have the potential to deprive us of the necessary building blocks which we require to build healthy connective tissue. In those with a predisposition to making poor quality connective tissue; this is not good news. The impact of a connective tissue disorder is widespread influencing the quality of life, earnings, relationships, among others.

Of course, genetically, there will always be an underlying predisposition to these conditions once you have been diagnosed with a connective tissue disorder such as EDS. You will always need to pay careful attention to your diet. This is no more than people, with other conditions, have to undertake on a daily basis. The patient is the best person to take control and responsibility for their condition.

Of course, I appreciate that people have different tastes; while introducing some foods into the diet will not cause any problems at all, some people may balk at some of them. This is not a problem. We can get around that. There are plenty of foods which contain the components needed to build healthy connective tissue. You just need to know what they are.

This book is intended to inform about the main building blocks of healthy connective tissue and how, by making a few simple changes to the diet, we can begin to ingest these necessary building blocks as a start to forming much stronger tissue.

As a result, you will develop stronger bones, ligaments and tendons. Your skin will be more elastic and younger looking and less prone to wrinkling. As a result of better formed connective tissue, your body will start to function better and pain should lessen.

Fortunately, it does not take long to build up a healthy gut lining or renew skin, tendons and ligaments and build up better bone. This begins to start immediately you provide the necessary building blocks although the full effects won't be felt for 30-45 days. However, one of the four main building blocks of cartilage has pain relieving properties and a marked reduction in pain can be felt within 24 hours. There have been many people who have emailed me to say that their pain has lessened, or disappeared - more or less overnight - and that they have been able to enjoy a proper night's sleep for the first time in years. This is how it should be. Pain is a warning that there is something wrong that needs to be addressed. It has no other function than that.

This book will show you how to harness the properties of these essential substances by changing your diet and/or supplementing where necessary. I think both are essential in the early stages since there is a lot of connective tissue repair that needs to be undertaken before the body goes into maintenance mode.

Please do not think that connective tissue disorders have a genetic basis and that there is nothing that can be done. This is nonsense; genes are turned on and off all the time by environmental influences; by far the greatest of these are the nutritional building blocks that you take into your body.

Cultural attitudes towards various foods are quite dynamic. As our eating patterns change, the amino acids that form the major part of our diet, change. An imbalance of amino acids will give rise to a susceptibility to specific disease states. The lack of amino acids which fuel the appearance of hypermobile conditions, are also responsible for pain syndromes, fibromyalgia, chronic fatigue syndrome, osteoarthritis and many others. Do these sound familiar? They should do since they are all disease states that currently afflict the majority of the developed population. Other 'popular' diseases have now slunk away and will only reappear if the amino acid balance – and its cofactors - is tipped in that direction once again. This is how important knowledge of nutrition is. Don't underestimate its power. It can change the course of a disease.

With all the hype that exists nowadays, do we eat a balanced diet? The truth is that we don't for we have removed some essential parts of an animal that provides nutrients in our diet that could ameliorate all the above conditions. Our focus, in this book, are they hypermobility syndromes. This is where we will begin, now.

Personal Journey

When I was a child, I was not aware of having any sort of connective tissue disorder at all (**CTD**). I had some problems with my joints but I was an active child so the pain was put down to that. I was given some foul smelling black ointment which, when rubbed into the skin, would change to olive green. That was quite fascinating but it did not stop the pain in my fingers or my thumb.

When I was a teenager I started getting shoulder pain. This was put down to the fact that I played the violin and my neck was in a strained position. However, when I stopped playing the violin, the pain didn't stop in my shoulders.

I was given Butazolidin which was a powerful anti-inflammatory. This didn't work all that well. Eventually, it was taken off the market and now it is just prescribed to horses.

Eventually, I was given Vioxx, but this too was taken off the market. The pain continued to flit about affecting various joints. My ankles were the main joints affected but I had constant back pain too, as well as recurring knee pain.

Even now, when I look at my toddler photos, my knees bend backwards. The photo on the page below shows the curve of my left leg but my right leg and knee also do this, too. I have since learned that this is called genu curvatum and is very common in hypermobility syndromes.

I never thought anything of it. It had always been like that. My legs were no different from that of my mother's legs and those of my siblings.

Ah yes, that is the side I inherited it from – my mother's side – although that wasn't quite the whole truth.

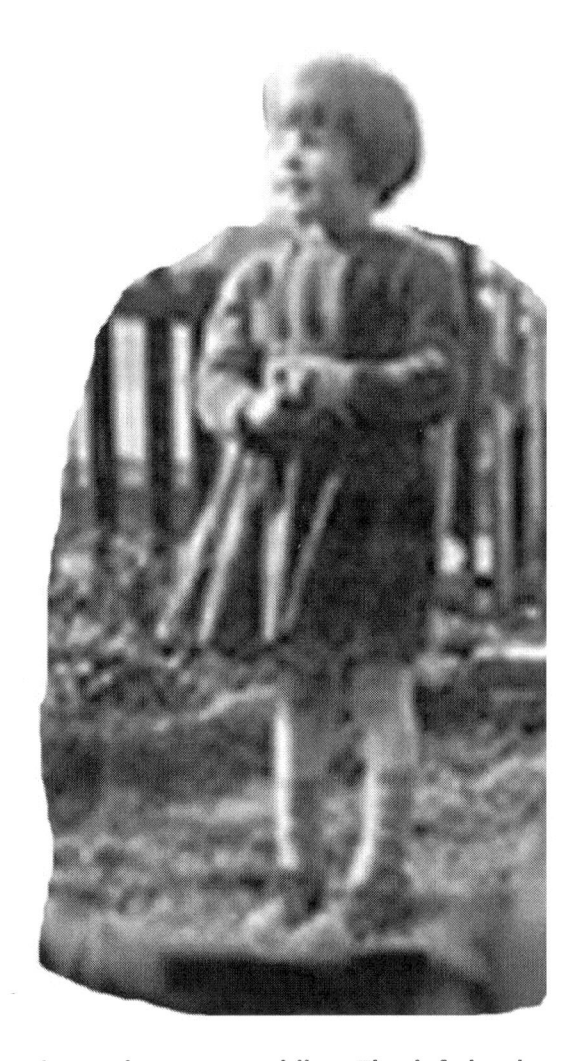

The author as a toddler. The left leg has a backwards curve (genu curvatum of -10)

My mother had similar legs. My mother could while bending over, keeping her legs straight, and placing her palms flat on the floor. I could also do that as well as place the thumb onto my same side wrist.

My mother had very wiggly toe joints. They run in the family and bend any way you can think of. At the time it was quite normal. I was a child; why would I think it would not be?

That was fun. I could actually do things that other children couldn't. Well, there was one school friend who could do that but we were definitely in the minority.

As I grew older I had unexplained bouts of tendonitis and back pain. I was active but so were many of my friends so that didn't explain why it kept happening to me. I spent a great deal of time off my feet, nursing swollen joints that I had done nothing to, apart from walk on.

Sometimes, my ankle would just 'give' and I couldn't put any weight on my foot for a few minutes. If I tried to pick up a pan with vegetables in, my wrist would also do the same.

It was painful and I had no prior warning when this was going to happen.

One day, I found that I could not get up the stairs. The act of lifting my foot up was so painful that I remained on the first step sobbing but unable to move either way. I was the mother of small children and I couldn't afford to be like this.

One day, I found that my ankle had blown up like a balloon. I hadn't sustained any injury. I hobbled to the Accident and Emergency unit where they were convinced I must have had an accident that I wasn't telling them about.

When I was out walking, my knees would bend backwards and throw me off balance. It would hurt and there was no telling when it would happen.

It continued like this. I was in pain most of the time and it became a part of me. I learned, almost subconsciously, not to do certain things. People thought I was being lazy. It wasn't laziness; it was self-preservation.

Hypermobility syndromes seem hard to detect by the medical profession even though the signs are all there. I did, on occasions, end up in the rheumatology department where it was recorded that my hypermobile knees had a score of -10. Nobody told me this. I only found this out when I was sifting through old medical records to see which ones I could throw away.

It doesn't take long to take a history of those who have persistent joint pain and ascertain whether other symptoms such as:

- **Joint pain and 'clicky' joints**
- **Heartburn and constipation and other digestive problems**
- **Fatigue**
- **Joint hypermobility**
- **Loose joints that dislocate quite easily**
- **Easy bruising**
- **PoTS – dizziness with increased heart rate after standing up**

but for unknown reasons it remains unrecognised and undiagnosed, for decades, in many people.

I am sure that it would have continued to be undiagnosed in me if it were not for the fact that a distance cousin contacted me. This was on the paternal side and her child had EDS. When we did a little digging, they weren't the only relatives we found that had a form of connective tissue disorder.

I had a challenge on my hands.

Collagen

Collagen is the most abundant protein to be found in the human body. It makes up about 30% of the protein to be found in the human body. It is found in:

- Bones
- Skin
- Muscles
- Tendons
- Ligaments
- The gut lining

Collagen is a protein which actually holds the body together. It acts like a scaffold strengthening and providing support.

Collagen helps to heal cartilage. Cartilage helps to cushion joints including the vertebrae which cause so much pain and suffering. Without properly synthesised collagen we would suffer recurring joint problems including dislocations, soft tissue injuries and gastro intestinal disturbances. Does this sound familiar?

Collagen is primarily made up of four amino acids. These are:

- Proline
- Hydroxyproline
- Arginine
- Glycine

We shall look at these in more detail in a little while.

Provided diets contain enough of the building blocks of collagen AND there aren't any genetic defects which would not support this, then the body will synthesise its own collagen. As it is synthesised within, it is known as *endogenous* collagen.

Exogenous collagen is collagen which is eaten through diets or supplementation. There are many such supplements on the market. They tend to be expensive and are generally made from the parts of animals which we throw away such as the chicken skin and the bones of animals as well as fish skin.

These parts of the animal were very much a part of the diets in the war and immediate post war years. The motto was:

Waste not, want not

No self-respecting housewife would throw away bones or fish heads before making a stock out of them. This was real flavoursome, healthy stock.

Now we thrown the carcase of a chicken away; we do not buy fish with the heads on so that we can use it later. Industry uses them though and they make good profit out of it.

These bits that are discarded are dried and powered before being sold as supplements with health giving properties.

The reality is that we throw away the very food that has the same health giving properties that we are prepared to buy later which is dried and packed in capsules.

It doesn't make sense really.

The supplements which are made from chicken skin and fish heads are full of gelatin.

Gelatin is the cooked form of collagen.

Gelatin contains about:

- 21% glycine
- 12% proline
- 12% hydroxyproline
- 8% arginine

We ingest very little of the above amino acids nowadays. When I was little, a chicken carcase was simmered to make bone broth or the fish

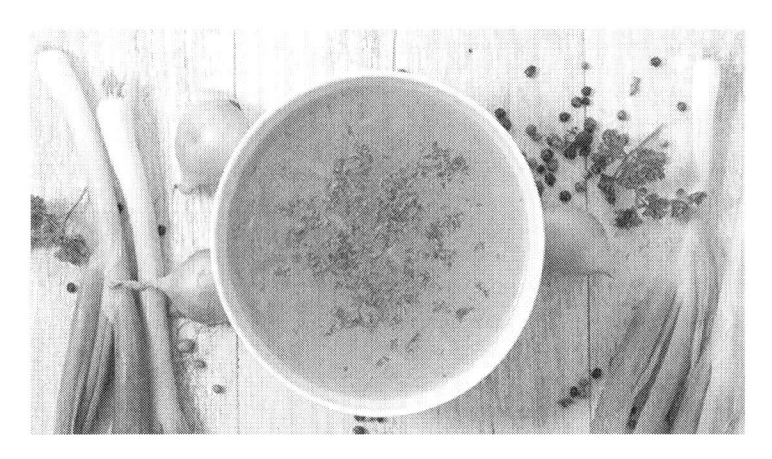

Bone broth is full of goodness[1]

heads put to one side to make soup. Tripe[2] was enjoyed sprinkled with a liberal amount of vinegar and eaten with gusto. These meals provided a goodly amount of the collagen forming amino acids.

Most of the amino acids found in diets nowadays are ones which increase stress and aging. That is, the muscle meats produce a stream of amino acids which reflect the combination of amino acids found when the

---

[1] https://recipes.mercola.com/turkey-bone-broth-recipe.aspx
[2] Tripe is a type of edible lining from the stomachs of various farm animals, generally cattle and sheep.

body is under extreme stress and muscle is broken down to provide energy to deal with it.

Glycine – the main amino acid in collagen - on the other hand is not generally found in the 'active' muscle meats. However, although it is the smallest amino acid, it has many important functions in the body.

Glycine is an inhibitory amino acid. It calms the brain down. As such, it acts as a pain reliever and it impacts on many of our functions. For example:

- It helps in the production of human growth hormone
- Produces bile salts and digestive enzymes
- Lowers inflammation
- Stabilises blood sugar and so is helpful in type 2 diabetes
- Boosts mental performance and energy
- Prevents the loss of cartilage in joints

Good things, do indeed, come in small packages.

In addition, it may help to reduce muscle wasting which occurs with aging – sarcopenia –

or malnutrition or when your body is under stress. Individual's with EDS and hypermobility syndromes are naturally wary of using limbs, given the propensity to dislocation or tendonitis, but this reluctance can also lead to further muscle wasting which, in turn, makes the joints even more vulnerable. Strong muscles help stabilise joints.

Although leucine, another amino acid, is generally credited with being the muscle building amino acid, it does not work well when the individual has wasting due to illness. It is here that glycine comes into its own. Research has shown that glycine was able to stimulate muscle growth during illness.[3]

Glycine works better in maintaining muscle mass in illness than leucine, normally credited with being the 'muscle building amino acid.

The pain found in connective tissue disorders can also be alleviated by consuming gelatin. Some of this gelatin will find its way into joint cartilage to help repair it, but this is not the process which alleviates the pain within a very

---
[3] https://www.ncbi.nlm.nih.gov/pubmed/27094036

short time of consumption. This incorporation of the components of gelatin into cartilage helps control pain over a longer period. It is glycine – found in the gelatin - that has inhibitory effects in the brain. These effects occur quite rapidly, soothing pain often more quickly than over the counter analgesics. Glycine also has an anti-inflammatory effect.

Glycine has pain relieving and anti-inflammatory effects.

Glycine can be bought online or in health food shops and up to 10g can be safely taken every day, for two weeks, in divided doses to control pain and/or to increase the amount of this collagen forming amino acid. After two weeks, the dose can be reduced to 3-5g daily.

Glycine is quite sweet and comes in crystalline form so can be used to sprinkle over cereal, on porridge, over fruit and incorporated into smoothies; indeed, anywhere where you would use sugar normally. It tastes great in coffee, for example.

Gelatin is colourless and flavourless and is normally bought to be used as a gelling agent. As such, it can be added to soups and stews to thicken them or added to yogurts or stewed fruit. You could also make your own home made fresh fruit jellies with gelatin.

10-15gms taken before bedtime can aid a full night's restful sleep. It can be added to a little water to soften, for a few minutes, before being added to a hot drink. If you try and add gelatin crystals straight into a hot drink, it will just form a sticky mass.

Gummy bears and wine gums are a couple of a wide range of sweets which are made from gelatin. Gelatin is also incorporated into marshmallows. Normally pork gelatin is used in these types of confectionary but there are vegetarian versions which you can obtain at your local supermarket.

However, before you rush to the sweet shop you might like to consider making bone broth which is full of health giving gelatin. I normally make bone broth from the carcases and skin of a chicken.

Bone Broth

Ingredients and method

One carcase of a chicken - include skin if this hasn't already been eaten. Place in the slow cooker with a few vegetables and black pepper, if desired. I add a pinch of herbs sometimes. Cover with water.

Add a squeeze of lemon juice. This helps calcium leach from the bones.

Cook on low/medium for 4-5 hours. Long slow cooking is essential if you want to extract the vital nutrients.

Drain the stock into a bowl and throw the bones and skin away. The stock will set as a gelatinous like substance eventually.

The stock is wonderful. It has antimicrobial properties and is full of gelatin. It makes a delicious base for soups and is perfect for risottos.

I have found that after drinking a cupful of this, my joint pain disappears. It gives a feeling of 'all is well with the world'. I actually prefer this to eating the chicken and make sure I have a good supply of this stock in the freezer at all times.

Although I normally use the chicken carcase, for making stock, any bones can be used. My favourite from the old days is oxtail which can be made in a similar way to the above. Just make sure that whenever bones come your way, that you don't throw them out before making a bone broth with them.

During the war years, nothing was wasted – even pigs' trotters could contribute to a warming gelatinous soup if they were slowly simmered for some time.

If a return to some of the recipes which were part of the daily diet in the 1940's and 1950's does not appeal – although I think you should give them a try - then there are plenty of collagen powders online which are made from dried fish scales, chicken feet, among others which you could add to shakes, omelettes or soups. There are also supplements of collagen available which are also convenient for those who do not enjoy cooking. 10-15g daily should suffice for those who have poor connective tissue.

Of course, if you have a sweet tooth then it is quite easy to make your own wine gums, too. Wine gums normally contain large quantities of glucose so making your own means that you can use natural unsweetened fruit juices, if that is your preference. If you prefer something a little sweeter then the liquid sweeteners come into their own here. Only a few drops are required. I add glycine to my wine gums although it is not as sweet as sugar.

Further benefits from glycine

Glycine makes glutathione which is one of the major antioxidants in the body. It combines with two other amino acids, cysteine and glutamate to make this important antioxidant.

Glutathione helps to combat free radicals which are molecules that can damage body cells.

Glutathione also helps to detoxify chemicals – free radicals - which have either been produced naturally in the body or are the result of pollutants in the environment.

Glycine helps to make an important antioxidant called glutathione

Glycine helps make creatine which helps to build:

- Muscle mass
- It has benefits for those with ALS in that it improved motor function, reduced muscle loss and extended survival rate by 17%[4]
- Reduces seizure activity
- Increases dopamine levels and is therefore useful in treating Parkinson's disease.

---

[4] https://www.ncbi.nlm.nih.gov/pubmed/10086395

- It may protect against muscle wasting in muscle wasting conditions such as muscular dystrophy.
- It may protect your liver from alcohol induced damage
- It may improve sleep quality
- It may improve heart health
- It helps promote recovery from strokes

Glycine is found mainly in:
- Low fat sesame flour
- Chicken skin
- Pork skin (crackling)
- Gelatin powder
- Dried egg whites
- bacon
- beef
- lamb
- cuttlefish

 Although glycine is a non-essential amino acid that can be produced from serine, it is not always made effectively, or in large enough quantities, by the body to cope with the demands of modern day living. As such, supplementation is recommended especially for those with any type of connective tissue disorder.

Serine is another non-essential amino acid. It is found in nuts such as almonds and walnuts, peanuts, eggs, meat, lentils, chickpeas and shellfish.

Nuts are a good source of serine which is a precursor to glycine.

I noticed many years ago that the retired people who still ate a lot of peanut butter, were free from arthritic knees. Peanut butter, of course was one of the mainstays of the diets of those who lived through, and immediately after, the Second World War. My husband still eats it by the spoonful, straight from the jar. He has never had any connective tissue problems, normally associated with older age, and is still able to kneel down without discomfort in spite of being seventy-five. None of his contemporaries are able to do this.

I looked into this a little further and found that those individuals with high glycine diets did not have joint problems, nor had they ever had tendonitis, strains and sprains in spite of leading quite active lives.

Proline is one of those amino acids that nobody seems to have heard about yet its contribution to the health of connective tissue disorders cannot be ignored.

Proline is another non-essential amino acid that has a number of functions including tissue repair and cellular regeneration. It forms part of the composition of collagen. More proline is required – and produced - at times of soft tissue injury, surgery or severe burns.

There is a high demand for proline whenever tissue damage occurs.

Further, proline keeps muscles and joints flexible, reduces sagging and thus keeps wrinkles at bay. This is particularly useful for those who spend a lot of time in the sun.

People who go on diets tend to lose some of the underlying structure of the skin. The softness and roundness of their skin appears to collapse a little. This phenomenon is very likely to be due to the lack of proline in the diet.

A lack of proline in the diet can be responsible for strains and tears in soft tissue and a poor rate of healing.

Strains and tears in soft tissue are often due to a lack of proline in the diet.

Proline also helps to prevent arteriosclerosis – hardening of the arteries – and assists in balancing blood pressure levels.

Proline also helps the body break down protein from worn out cells in the body. This protein is further used to create new healthy cells. It is also required to form hydroxyproline another amino acid which is a major component of the protein, collagen.

Good sources of proline are:
- egg yolks
- grass fed meats
- organ meats – for example, liver and kidney.

- bone broth
- gelatin

If we look at the above foods in the light of our current eating preferences, grass fed meats, organ meats, bone broth and gelatin are foods of the past. Further, eggs have been demonised as being a contributory factor to high cholesterol levels. They may well be, but high cholesterol levels are associated with a number of healthy states and are associated with good health. This will be the subject of a later book.

Proline is made from glutamic acid. As long as the diet is sufficient in glutamic acid then there should be sufficient proline for individual needs. However, in cases of connective tissue disorder, it would be helpful to supplement with proline. We cannot discount that the process - by which proline is synthesised from glutamic acid – is malfunctioning and that this has contributed to poor tissue formation. By providing proline directly, in supplement form, we are bypassing one potentially missing – but essential – step that is required for collagen formation.

Be guided by the dosage instructions which accompanies this amino acid on its packaging. It is harder to find sources of proline than glycine and it does tend to be more expensive than glycine. However, it is worth sourcing, even if it is a one off purchase in order to see how effective supplementing with proline is in ameliorating the symptoms of hypermobile joints.

Glutamic acid, from which proline is made is found in all types of animal protein – eggs, meat, fish, cheese, for example, and does not usually need to be supplemented. However, if the diet needs supplementing at times of illness or advancing age then whey protein is an easily digestible source of all the essential amino acids.

Free form amino acids, if you can source them, do not need digesting. They are absorbed immediately.

About 30% of the protein in wheat is made from glutamic acid.

Vegetarian sources of proline include:
- cabbage
- peanuts
- soy products
- watercress
- asparagus
- white mustard seeds

Hydroxyproline

Hydroxyproline is a major component of the protein collagen. It helps to prevent fine lines and wrinkles found in aged or sun damaged skin.

Rat studies[5] found that there was an increasing effect of an oral intake of L-hydroxyproline on the soluble collagen content of skin.

In this study either 0.5 or 1g/kg of L-hydroxyproline (Hyp) was given to rats. After 2 weeks, administration of Hyp the soluble collagen content of the skin had increased.

---

[5] https://www.ncbi.nlm.nih.gov/pubmed/22790956

This suggested that oral Hyp, improved collagen metabolism.

Oral hydroxyproline improves the metabolism of collagen.

Any defect in collagen synthesis can lead to a number of effects such as easy bruising, breakdown of connective tissue, internal bleeding, thin walled blood vessels. As can be seen from the table below, without an adequate supply of vitamin C, then the synthesis of collagen, from hydroxyproline, cannot occur.

Vitamin C is a water soluble vitamin. It is found in fresh fruit and vegetables. It is easily destroyed by heat and sunlight.

The recommended daily allowance is 30mg daily which is the amount found in an orange. However, in connective tissue disorders, I would be recommending much higher amounts. There are some dissolving vitamin C tablets (ascorbic acid) which are generally a reasonable price. These can be found in supermarkets. They contain 1000mg of vitamin C. I would recommend four weeks of this high dose, a further four weeks of 500mg and following on from that, 100mg daily.

These 1000mg dissolvable tablets do contain high amounts of salt so an alternative should be sought in cases of an individual having high blood pressure. There are plenty of alternatives on the market.

As vitamin C is a water soluble tablet, any excess not required by the body is simply lost through urine.

There is little point in increasing vitamin c, though, if the proline content of food has not increased, too; both are required to make hydroxyproline.

Diagram showing chain of events in forming collagen from glutamic acid.

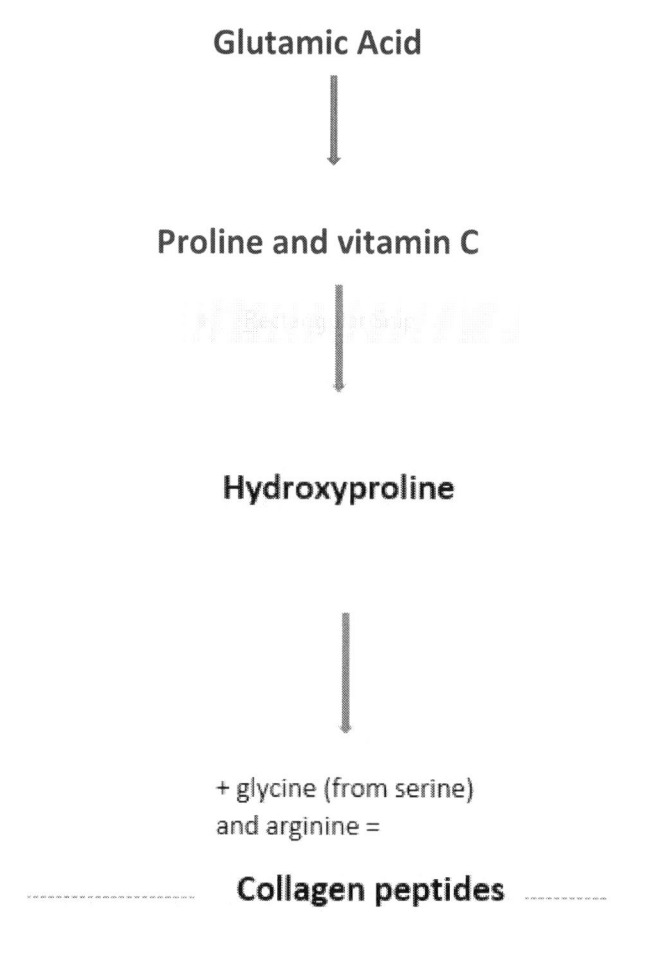

Glutamic Acid
↓

Proline and vitamin C
↓

Hydroxyproline
↓

+ glycine (from serine) and arginine =

Collagen peptides

Vegetarian and non-vegetarian sources of hydroxyproline

Non-vegetarian	Vegetarian
meat, pigs trotters,	carob seeds
eggs	Alfalfa sprouts
monkfish	Citrus fruits (or anything high in vitamin C)
eggs	Vegetable foods high in vitamin c (peppers, cabbage, parsley
Milk and dairy products	Non citrus fruits such as banana also help in the synthesis of hydroxyproline.
Shark cartilage	

.

Now that we have looked at glycine, proline and hydroxyproline, we will turn our attention to the fourth major component of collagen. This is the amino acid, arginine.

Arginine

Arginine is an essential amino acid which means that it has to be obtained from the diet. It is unusual in that, in the body, it is known to change into nitric oxide. Nitric oxide is a powerful neurotransmitter. It helps blood vessels to relax thereby improving circulation.

Arginine is also a component of many connective tissues and supports the production of collagen. Further, arginine assists with the growth of osteoblasts which are the cells which form bone mass.

A study[6] from 2002 showed that arginine was important for bone health since a deficiency of this amino acid was implicated in osteoporosis.

---

[6] https://www.aminoacid-studies.com/areas-of-use/arthritis-and-osteoporosis.html

A standard daily dose for arginine has not yet been agreed but most people ingest between 2-3 gms per day.

Good food sources of arginine are:

- turkey (one turkey breast contains about 16gm)
- pork loin (approximately 13gm)
- chicken
- peanuts
- soybeans
- dairy

When we are looking at the foods which contribute to healthy connective tissue then time and again the humble peanut turns up.

If you are a fan of peanuts and peanut butter then this is to your advantage but, of course, there are many people who have developed an allergy to the nuts in this spread. Allergies do appear rife in connective tissue disorders. However, the point that needs underlining is that peanuts are another food which was very popular during the war and immediate post war period and appears to have now fallen out of popularity along with many foods which promote the synthesis of healthy connective tissue.

However, the bone broth is still an essential for good connective tissue health. Add some garlic and onion to it and you are increasing the amount of methionine – another amino acid – which is required to build good cartilage.

Methionine is a sulphur containing amino acid. It helps to make SAM (S-adenosyl methionine) which is used in the production of creatine. This is an important substance for cellular energy.

Eggs, fish and meat contain good amounts of this amino acid.

Here are some recipes which will help increase those components required for good collagen synthesis.

Some people may think it is a lot of work making their own stock from bones and fish head and storing it in the freezer but it is definitely worth doing. The alternative is to use those stock cubes which contain mainly salt, a little yeast and some animal fat. The gelatin is absent and it is this we are trying to put back into the diet.

The stock will keep well for a month or so, in the freezer, but I never find it lasts that long. I always seem to have some on the go. I am quite happy throwing some bones into the slow cooker with some herbs, garlic and onion, waiting until it cools then transferring it to a jam jar before freezing it.

I leave about one-inch space to allow for expansion at the top of the jar.

When I eventually thaw the stock, it is entirely up to me what other vegetables I throw into it. I will add white wine to white meat and fish stocks and red wine to the darker meats and oilier fishes but really, all you need is a little motivation and a lot of imagination to produce your own range of tasty medicines.

In the words of the old adage:

Let food be your medicine

The role of zinc in connective tissue synthesis, maintenance and repair

Zinc is a vital nutrient that is involved in over 80 body processes. It is the second most abundant mineral to be found in the body. It is classed as an essential nutrient; It must be obtained through food, or supplements, on a daily basis as the body cannot make it by itself.

The array of processes that zinc has in your body is numerous. They include

- Gene expression
- Immune function – aids the development and function of immune cells
- Protein synthesis
- DNA synthesis
- Growth and development
- Wound healing – regulates inflammation and the production of new skin cells

Fortunately, zinc is found in a wide variety of foods but it is also added to foods that do not naturally contain zinc such as flour.

Zinc plays an essential role in collagen synthesis. About 5% of the total amount of zinc in your body is to be found in the skin.

Zinc is required for protein synthesis and the production of connective tissues such as bone and cartilage.

As zinc is found mainly in animal foods, individuals who follow a vegetarian or vegan diet are likely to be zinc deficient. As such, those individuals who do not eat animal protein and who have a connective tissue disorder, need to consider whether a zinc deficiency is the cause of it.

The recommended daily intake of zinc for an adult male is 9.5mg.

The recommended daily intake of zinc for an adult female is 7mg.

The Foods Standards Agency (UK) recommends no more than 25 mg daily.

Table Selected Food Sources of Zinc

Food	Milligrams (mg) per serving	Percent DV*
Oysters, cooked, breaded and fried, 3 ounces	74.0	493
Beef chuck roast, braised, 3 ounces	7.0	47
Crab, Alaska king, cooked, 3 ounces	6.5	43
Beef patty, broiled, 3 ounces	5.3	35
Breakfast cereal, fortified with 25% of the DV for zinc, ¾ cup serving	3.8	25
Lobster, cooked, 3 ounces	3.4	23
Pork chop, loin, cooked, 3 ounces	2.9	19
Baked beans, canned, plain or vegetarian, ½ cup	2.9	19
Chicken, dark meat, cooked, 3 ounces	2.4	16
Yogurt, fruit, low fat, 8 ounces	1.7	11
Cashews, dry roasted, 1 ounce	1.6	11
Chickpeas, cooked, ½ cup	1.3	9
Cheese, Swiss, 1 ounce	1.2	8
Oatmeal, instant, plain, prepared with water, 1 packet	1.1	7
Milk, low-fat or non fat, 1 cup	1.0	7
Almonds, dry roasted, 1 ounce	0.9	6
Kidney beans, cooked, ½ cup	0.9	6
Chicken breast, roasted, skin removed, ½ breast	0.9	6
Cheese, cheddar or mozzarella, 1 ounce	0.9	6
Peas, green, frozen, cooked, ½ cup	0.5	3
Flounder or sole, cooked, 3 ounces	0.3	2

7

---

[7] https://ods.od.nih.gov/factsheets/Zinc-HealthProfessional/

Reasonable vegetarian sources of zinc are:

- Fortified cereals
- Wheat germ
- Lentils
- Yogurt
- Oatmeal
- Wild rice
- Hemp seeds
- Tofu
- Wild rice
- Milk and
- Squash seeds
- Beans
- nuts

Even so, you may have to consider zinc supplements if you are vegan or vegetarian since none of the above contain inspiring amounts of zinc.

Other common symptoms of zinc deficiency include:

- increased rates of diarrhoea
- eczema
- seborrheic dermatitis
- acne
- impaired wound healing
- alopecia
- increased susceptibility to respiratory infections such as pneumonia
- gastrointestinal infections

Tendons and the amino acids

The basic function of the tendon is to transfer the force initiated by the muscle to the bone. This allows joint movement.

Tendons have to be tough as they are exposed to forces from all directions. They are composed mainly of the protein collagen but they also consist of a small amount of elastin.

Elastin is a highly elastic protein in connective tissue. This is the protein that helps the tissues in the body to resume their shape after being stretched or contracted. If you push your skin in, gently, on your abdomen then it will return to its original position due to the elastin in it. This phenomenon can be understood when we think of the expansion and contraction of the lungs or the bladder.

The amino acids that make up elastin are:

- glycine
- alanine
- valine
- proline

We have already looked at glycine and proline so we will turn our attention to alanine and valine now.

Alanine

Alanine is a small non-essential amino acid in humans. It is classed as non-essential as the body is supposed to be able to make it from other substances. However, sometimes this mechanism is faulty and the aging process is not as effective in assisting the transformation of amino acids that occurs when younger.

Alanine helps the synthesis of proteins from various amino acids, especially tryptophan which is a calming amino acid. It also helps to synthesise the vitamin pyridoxine most commonly known as vitamin B6.

Vitamin B6 is important for healthy hair, skin and nerves.

The foods highest in alanine are fish and meat. There is some to be found in soya and lima beans but again, a vegan or vegetarian diet is unlikely to provide enough of this amino acid.

Valine

Valine is an amino acid that is important for assisting in everyday bodily functions. It helps to regulate the immune system and build muscles. Many amino acids are processed by the liver but in valine's case, it is immediately used by the muscles. It is therefore, a good source of immediate energy.

Good sources of valine are:

- Poultry
- Milk
- Leafy vegetables
- Kidney beans

Finally, we should not forget the role of **leucine**, an essential amino acid that directly stimulates muscle growth and repair. Leucine has also been found to stimulate tendon formation. In addition, it slows down the passage of pain signals to the nervous system.

Where do we find leucine? Leucine is found in animal protein especially chicken, turkey and fish, dairy products like cheese and yogurt and soybeans.

There are smaller amounts in nuts, seeds, eggs and fruit.

To look at the difference in the elasticity of the skin of someone with enough elastin, gently pull the skin, on the back of the hand, of a young person and compare it with that of someone of middle age or older. The skin of an older person does not snap back to its original shape so readily. This should provide the impetus to increase the amino acids that form elastin.

In fact, any of the 'stretchy' confectionary like wine gums, midget gems, marshmallows, 'milk bottles' and other gums are generally made with gelatin and will contain the amino acids found in the protein, elastin. As a treat they are the preferred form over other traditional sweets for individuals with a connective tissue disorder or the older person whose skin has lost some elasticity.

We often forget that poor synthesis of connective tissue doesn't just end with the outward appearance. Blood vessels, organs and ligaments also contain elastin. It is found throughout the body. The skin just reflects the amount of elastin found in the above. If your skin is in a poor state then your organs, blood vessels, ligaments and tendons will not be functioning properly either. This needs rectifying for optimum health.

Other nutrients involved in connective tissue synthesis

Glucosamine Sulphate

There are some studies that suggest that orally administered glucosamine sulphate normalises cartilage metabolism by stimulating proteoglycan synthesis. Proteoglycans are found in connective tissue and its composition is gel like thus accounting for the high compressibility of cartilage.

Glucosamine is found in good quantities in bone broth.

Vitamin C

Although I have already mentioned vitamin C its role in collagen fibre synthesis cannot be underlined enough. A deficiency of vitamin C is associated with poor collagen formation and delayed wound healing.

The American Journal of Clinical Nutrition (issue one, January 2017, pages 136-143) cites research that shows that vitamin C enriched gelatin supplementation augments collagen synthesis.

In their introduction this journal reports:

The structure and function of musculoskeletal tissues, such as tendon, ligaments, cartilage and bone, are dependent on their collagen rich extracellular matrix. This matrix, in turn, derives its function from the amount and the crosslinking of this collagen together with the water or mineral within the tissue. In disease states or in the presence of a nutritional or genetic insufficiency, a poor extracellular matrix is produced that is unable to withstand the mechanical demands of normal activity.

While poor nutrition, genetics and disease can make connective tissue prone to failure, adequate nutrition together with exercise normally improves the function of the matrix. Acute exercise is known to increase collagen synthesis as well as the expression of the primary enzyme involved in collagen crosslinking, lysil oxidase. The result is a denser and stiffer tissue after training that is stronger.

Copper

Lysil oxidase is a copper enzyme that is involved in the cross linking of elastin and collagen. As such it is necessary for proper collagen formation and maintenance.

When a copper deficiency occurs then damaged connective tissue cannot be replaced. Further, the collagen that makes up the scaffolding of the bone cannot be formed leading to a condition known as osteoporosis.

Foods which contain copper include:

- Liver
- Oysters
- Nuts and seeds
- Lobster
- Dark leafy greens
- Dark chocolate

The recommended dietary allowance is 900mcg daily. However, a word of caution is required here – a deficiency or excess of copper can have negative side effects so supplementation is not recommended unless under medical supervision. My recommendation is that every individual with a connective tissue disorder, such as EDS, look at the composition of their diet to ascertain if it contains any foods that contain copper and to include them if they are sparse.

The following foods are excellent sources of copper:[8]

	Amount	RDI
Beef liver, cooked	1 oz (28 g)	458%
Oysters, cooked	6	133%
Lobster, cooked	1 cup (145 g)	141%
Lamb liver, cooked	1 oz (28 g)	99%
Squid, cooked	3 oz (85 g)	90%
Dark chocolate	3.5 oz bar (100 g)	88%
Oats, raw	1 cup (156 g)	49%
Sesame seeds, roasted	1 oz (28 g)	35%
Cashew nuts, raw	1 oz (28 g)	31%

---

[8] https://www.healthline.com/nutrition/copper-deficiency-symptoms#section11

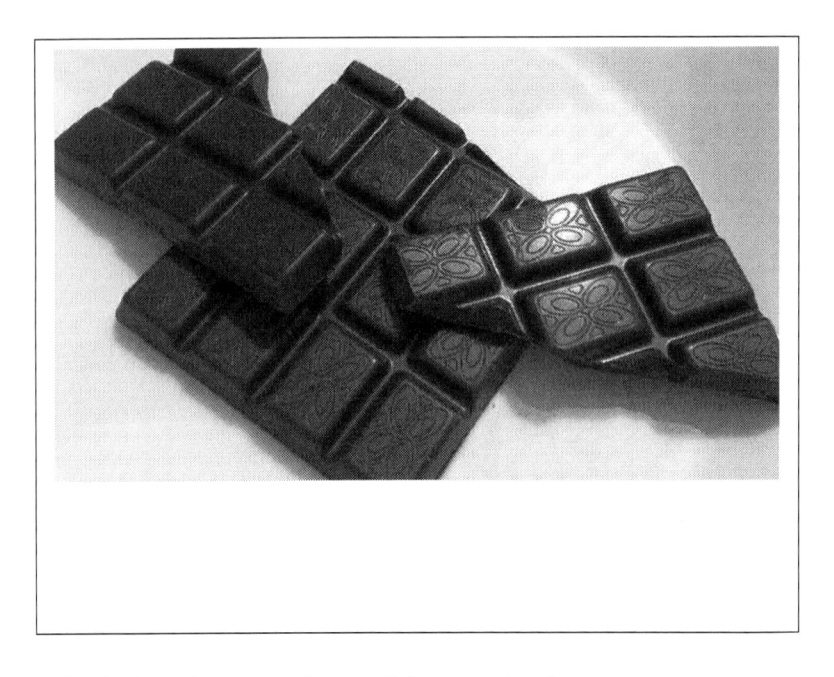

Dark chocolate contains useful amounts of copper

Foods which contain high amounts of zinc are:

- Legumes
- Meat
- Dairy
- Nuts
- Seeds
- Whole grains
- Eggs

Bioflavonoids

Bioflavonoids are substances found in plants. They have a potential role in relieving pain as they inhibit enzymes such as:

- Lipoxygenase
- Phospholipase
- Prostaglandin cyclooxygenase

Prostaglandin cyclooxygenase is an enzyme that helps to make prostaglandins. Some prostaglandins are known to induce elastase – an enzyme that breaks down elastin. Bioflavonoids appear to bind to elastin preventing its breakdown.

Prostaglandin cyclooxygenase form
⇩
Prostaglandins which help induce
⇩
Elastase which breaks down

Elastin which is

A NECESSARY COMPONENT OF CONNECTIVE TISSUE

BIOFLAVANOIDS STOP THE BREAKDOWN OF ELASTIN

Elastases are released as a result of inflammation therefore it stands to reason that anything that reduces inflammation will help collagen formation.

Bioflavonoids also help to activate some enzymes most noticeably that of proline hydroxylase which is necessary for collagen cross linking.

Bioflavonoids are found in the array of multi-coloured fruit and vegetables that we are encouraged to eat as part of a healthy diet.

Some Observations

During my time talking with people who have various forms of EDS it has become increasingly apparent that their symptoms often initially became noticeable after periods in their lives when nutritional needs were sadly neglected – often during young adulthood. Some of the deficiencies that were the result of poor eating habits such as vitamin D and iron deficiency anaemia, were addressed by the medical establishment at the time. These are standard tests in the UK. They are easy to administer and the results are fairly conclusive. The remedies are also easy to administer in a cost effective manner. However, when nutritional status has been poor, for whatever reason, it is highly probable that deficiencies of many other vital nutrients will be missed and not addressed. Tests for these may not be routinely available for a number of reasons. Some may be difficult to administer, for example, and others not sensitive enough to provide conclusive proof of a specific deficiency.

If nutritional deficiencies continue to remain unaddressed then they cannot do anything but impact on some part of the body. In connective tissue disorders a number, but finite, amount of nutritional deficiencies can contribute to the varying connective tissue disorders that are rife in society at the moment. It may well be that a lack of one specific nutrient – or a specific mix of vital nutrients involved in connective tissue synthesis - may account for one of the recognised types of connective tissue disorder. The vascular EDS, for example, may partially occur as a result of insufficient dietary copper necessary to make copper enzymes which are vital for the cross linking of elastin and collagen.

In cases such as these, correcting an iron deficiency anaemia and vitamin D deficiency, that has been revealed through standard medical tests, may alleviate some associated disease states but they are unlikely to address any connective tissue disease states that have occurred through poor nutrition. If this lack of specific attention to good nutrition continues then the medical condition will also continue to worsen carrying with it the promise of further and increasing debilitating illness.

When I have examined the contents of the formula fed to those with EDS who are tube fed, I am struck that an overall recommended day's supply - that should contain all the nutrients to build up the entire body and maintain its processes - hardly contains half of what is required for the building up and maintenance of the human body, including connective tissue. Is this not slow starvation? It is not difficult to see how this illness degenerates when there is not enough of the vital nutritional substances available to make good connective tissue.

For too long I have heard that EDS has a genetic basis and therefore nothing can be done about it. However, while there may be a genetic propensity to certain disease states they do not exist in isolation from environmental factors and environmental factors have the greatest sway in these matters. Nutrition is unarguably powerful and those with EDS and hypermobility syndromes need to be educated on the composition of connective tissue –as do many in the medical profession – so that they can address the nutritional deficiencies in their diet. This may be achieved with the help of a dietician with a special interest in connective tissue disorders.

Some further considerations

When anyone has a disease state, they have to be prepared to take responsibility for that condition. In many cases this may mean adjusting the diet to accommodate the deficiencies or excesses that have led to the symptoms in the first place.

With the hypermobility disease states, this is a fairly straightforward process if you do not like cooking. I find it therapeutic but I recognise that not everyone feels the same.

If you are one of those people who balk at the thought of making bone broth then the easy way is to simply sprinkle gelatin on your food, add a good multi vitamin supplement and add some whey protein, egg white and powdered milk to your food. That's the easy way out for those who don't have time or don't like cooking.

However, food deserves a healthy respect. Food is medicine and the more you incorporate what you have learned here, the more you will be armed to take control of your medical condition by changing around your diet to accommodate your state of health. As I have already mentioned our current healthy eating patterns are not really healthy given that they have excluded many of the smaller amino acids that are essential for the composition of healthy connective tissue.

You need to learn about nutrition. It is too important to be relegated to the odd glance at a newspaper article on an obscure super food. Once you have absorbed the information in this book, start creating your own recipes that will help incorporate the amino acids that are required for healthy connective tissue into delicious meals.

I generally suggest that before embarking on this new way of eating that you take a photograph and a further one 45 days later. You should find a marked improvement in your skin, I also suggest that you take a mental note of your pain levels on the day that you embark on this new way of eating and also when they drop rapidly. Glycine has this effect. It is a marvellous amino acid.

Tendons and ligaments take longer to form optimally once the correct balance of nutrients is ingested. However, the process **starts** from the moment they are ingested.

To give you some idea of how you can incorporate the amino acids that are important in hypermobility syndromes, I have included some recipes below to help you get started.

Recipes

Risotto

Ingredients

- 4 ounces of Arborio rice per person for the main meal or 2 ounces per person for a starter.
- Bone broth stock – approximately three times as much as the rice
- A knob of butter
- Finely chopped vegetables – mushrooms, tomatoes, peas, onions, for example, to taste
- Protein source to 'match' the stock source. For example, fish if using fish source.

- A little white wine if desired – stock and wine can be used half and half of each.
- Extra stock may be required.

Method

Add the chopped vegetables and protein source, if meat, to the melted butter in the pan and sauté extremely gently for two minutes.

Fish should be added towards the end of the cooking time if your protein source is fish and not meat.

Add the rice and sauté gently for a minute then add a ladleful of the liquid broth or wine/stock mix.

Keep stirring on a gentle simmer until all the liquid is practically absorbed, then add another ladleful.

Keep doing this until all the liquid has been added and has absorbed.

The rice should look creamy.

Test to see that it is soft. It should have been cooking for about 20-25 minutes. If it requires a little longer then add a little more stock or wine until the desired texture is reached.

Peanut satay

Ingredients

- one tablespoon of coconut oil
- one clove of crushed garlic
- one small chilli and one small onion chopped
- 2 tablespoons of peanut butter (your choice of whether crunchy or smooth)
- 200 mls of coconut milk

Method

Gently fry the garlic, chilli and onion in the coconut oil.

Stir in the peanut butter and coconut milk until it forms a paste.

I use this in a stir fry or I cook chicken, add the satay sauce and serve over egg noodles or rice. Some people add soy sauce to the satay but I think it is just as nice without.

Fruit cups

Ingredients

Pureed fruit of choice (about two cups full and one tablespoon of gelatin).

Method

Soften the gelatin in a little of the fruit puree. Warm the rest of the fruit puree in the pan. It doesn't have to boil but it does need to be warm enough for the gelatin to be able to dissolve in it.

When the gelatin has dissolved, add it all to the warm puree and stir until it has dissolved.

At this stage you can add sweetening agent if that is your preference. I generally use glycine because it is sweet and one of the major components of collagen, anyway.

Pour into cups and let the fruit cups set in the refrigerator.

Shepherd's pie

This is actually made with organ meats and was one of my children's favourites when they were little. I simply cooked the liver and onions slowly, with a little water and a stock cube, and then I minced it in the food processor, layered it in a dish before topping with potato or a mix of root vegetables.

It is a much cheaper version of our Shepherd's Pie and contains more of the nutrients required for connective tissue health than the usual lamb mince.

Fish Head Soup

Ingredients

- One tablespoon of oil
- One onion
- One chopped carrot
- One stalk of celery chopped
- Some parsley
- Half teaspoon of fennel seeds
- A bay leaf
- 200mls of tinned tomatoes
- Chopped garlic to taste
- 200mls of white wine
- 2ib of fish heads, skeleton and skin. Remove the gills as they impart a bitter flavour.

- **Method**

Gently fry the onion, carrot, celery, fennel seeds and garlic in the oil. Add the other ingredients and simmer for no longer than 15 minutes. Lay on one side to cool. Once cool transfer the whole lot to the refrigerator until the following day. This allows the flavours to develop.

Strain, heat gently and serve.

To give it extra substance, you can add cooked rice or eat with cheese on toast.

Chinese soup

Ingredients

- One litre of chicken stock made from simmering bones
- Diced chicken – about 2-4 ounce per person

- Chinese five spice to taste
- Fresh ginger chopped – about one inch
- Shredded pak choi
- Chopped onion
- Chopped tomato
- Sweetcorn
- Fennel chopped
- Mushrooms – half to be diced and the other half to be sliced and gently fried
- Seasoning as desired
- A little oil for frying

Method

Fry the diced chicken, onion, tomato, five spice, chopped tomato. sweetcorn and diced mushrooms gently for 3-4 minutes, stirring continuously.

Add the stock and simmer for ten minutes until the chicken is cooked through.

Quickly add the seasoning, the fresh ginger, pack choi and fennel. Turn off the heat and allow to stand for two minutes before serving with the sliced mushrooms served on the top of the soup.

Chick Pea and Bean Curry (vegetarian)

Ingredients

- 2 onions – one diced, one sliced
- One tablespoon of oil
- Chopped garlic cloves to taste
- Fresh root ginger
- A fresh chilli or dried chilli to taste (about one teaspoonful)
- Two tablespoons of curry powder
- A can of mixed beans
- A can of chickpeas
- A can of tomatoes
- Green leafy veg. For example, diced spinach or diced chard.

- A dollop of mango chutney or a teaspoonful of sugar
- Seasoning – pepper or salt to taste

Method

Place all the ingredients in the slow cooker and cook on a low heat for 3-4 hours which will allow all the flavours to mingle.

Note: although the beans do provide **glycine,** it is not enough for an individual's needs especially if they have a connective tissue disorder.

Please see link below for a useful table showing the main vegetarian sources of glycine.

With regards to **proline**, practically all the main sources of proline are from complete protein sources. The precursor of proline is glutamic acid and there is usually plenty of this amino acid in our current preferred eating patterns. Nevertheless, proline deficiency is not unusual in both meat eaters, and non- meat eaters. It may be that something goes wrong in the conversion of proline from glutamic acid. We already know that proline needs to be taken with vitamin C in order for it to be converted to hydroxyproline.

Conversion from one amino acid to another generally requires at least one co-factor – and often more than one – for this to be undertaken successfully.

Proline – the main sources are:

Dried egg white – 3200mg per 100g

Swiss cheese – 2750mg per 100g

Dried milk powder - 3500 per 100g

Mustard seed - 2750 mg per 100g

Vegetarian sources of gelatin
- Agar agar – use the same amount of agar-agar as you would gelatin
- Carrageenan (Irish Moss) – use one ounce to each cupful of fluid. Boil for ten minutes and then strain the carrageenan.

Please note that vegetarian sources of gelatin may be used to set food but this does not mean

that they contain the same amino acids as animal gelatin which is essential for healthy connective tissue.

Plant based sources of glycine

(but unfortunately plants sources only contain small amounts of glycine)
- Beans
- Cauliflower
- Cabbage
- Spinach
- Kale
- Peanuts

Link to vegetarian sources of glycine

https://nutritiondata.self.com/foods-011094000000000000000-1.html

As we have now examined the main amino acids that connective tissue is composed of then it would be prudent to turn our attention to a hormone that is vital for the production of collagen. When we consider how much the health of connective tissue is impacted from various sources, the more that we understand that eating a diversity of foods supports the optimum function of connective tissue.

Progesterone deficiency and its role in the synthesis of healthy connective tissue

Progesterone is a hormone that is generally made in the ovaries but lesser amounts are made in the adrenal glands and the placenta. Progesterone receptors have been found on connective tissue which is why the importance of progesterone to connective tissue was established.

Rececptors are proteins which sit on the surface of a cell. These receptor proteins receive a chemical signal from progesterone, in this particular example. However, there are receptors for every single vitamin, mineral and any other substances found in the body. The importance of these to any specific organ and tissue is highlighted by the presence of specific receptors.

Receptors, when bound to their ligand, initiate responses which can regulate various processes or induce cell growth, division or death depending on what substance they are affiliated to.

Progesterone regulates the activity of collagenase which is an enzyme that breaks down the peptide bonds in collagen. This allows a balance between production and degradation.

Progesterone is vital for the production of collagen. It helps to increase the elasticity and thickness of skin.

There are many causes of low progesterone. This condition is not just related to the ageing process. Excess weight will tip the balance in favour of oestrogen dominance. Further, stress will transform progesterone, through action by the kidneys to the stress hormone cortisol.

Surprisingly, low cholesterol may also contribute hypo-progesterone. The precursor to progesterone is another hormone called pregnenolone. Cholesterol is required for the synthesis of pregnenolone and other hormones. When cholesterol levels are inadequate, then vital hormones cannot be synthesised. In some cases, the synthesis of hormones may be impacted by statins.

Although there are a number of creams which can be rubbed into the skin and are said to raise progesterone levels, many of these contain a substance known as diosgenin. Diosgenin is extracted from the wild yam. However, the human body cannot make progesterone from diosgenin only pregnenolone.

Pregnenolone is a steroid that is made within the brain, gonads and adrenal glands. It is made from cholesterol. Most cholesterol is made and regulated in the body. A small amount is obtained from animal foods such as meat and full fat dairy foods. A little is mad from fats found in olive oil and avocados. Lowering cholesterol through the use of medication may hamper the synthesis of vital hormones. Pregnenolone is the precursor to many steroid hormones including the:

- Progestogens
- Eostrogens
- Androgens
- Glucocorticoids

- mineralcorticoids

Diet can also affect the production of progesterone. Magnesium and vitamin B6 both boost progesterone levels. Indeed, research has shown that high vitamin B6 levels reduce the chance of miscarriage by 50% as well as increasing fertility by 120% through the synthesis of progesterone. Optimum levels of progesterone are required for the continuation of the pregnancy.

Vitamin B6 is an essential co-factor required for the normal speed of the cross linking of collagen by enzymes. The strength of collagen is partially dependent on this vitamin.

The importance of making sure that you have adequate magnesium levels needs to be underlined. Magnesium is required for the synthesis of collagen and elastin as well as the breakdown of worn out collagen and elastin.

In younger women, optimum levels of zinc increase the level of follicle stimulating hormone (FSH). Once FSH reaches optimum levels ovulation will occur. After ovulation has occurred the ovaries will make progesterone to prepare the uterus for a potential pregnancy.

Vitamin C is the king of vitamins when it comes to raising progesterone levels. Studies have shown that high levels had a significant impact on progesterone levels, increasing the amount by 77% when 750mg were taken daily.

When you consider that the daily recommended amount of vitamin C is 60 mg you can see that this amount is hopelessly inadequate. In fact, this amount was recommended as a sufficient daily intake as it prevented the deficiency disease scurvy. However, although it may prevent scurvy it does not promote optimum health. It is the very minimum that you can get away with in order to maintain life.

Beta carotene is also able to stimulate production of progesterone. Beta carotene is the precursor to vitamin A. Many orange coloured vegetables such as carrots and pumpkin contain good amounts of beta carotene.

Further, vitamin E is able to stimulate production. 150 IU's has been mooted as providing the best benefits. Intakes higher than this may actually be counterproductive. Vitamin E is found in nuts and wheat germ, mainly.

It can be seen that inadequate levels of essential vitamins, macro and trace minerals may contribute to low progesterone levels thus increasing the potential for poor quality connective tissue .

Books in the EDS Series

Alleviating Symptoms of EDS – addresses gastroparesis and other digestive problems, pain and sleep problems (published August 2019)

The EDS Diet Recipe book

The Journey: living with EDS and chronic pain

The EDS and Hypermobility Syndrome Diet

Causes of Weight Gain in EDS (published July 2020)

05/05/19 I am pleased to say that my latest book The EDS Recipe Book is now published and available to buy online in paperback and on Kindle. This is a further step forward in helping people to change their eating habits in order to form healthy connective tissue as many of the nutrients which do this are no longer a regular part of our diets. These recipes are simple to make and often include our old favourites but with an additional twist. These recipes are also just as useful for people with osteoarthritis - a condition that is often an outcome of having a condition like EDS or hypermobility syndrome.

Thank you for purchasing this book.

Every time a book is purchased, a donation is made to one of the charities I am currently supporting. These can be found on the author's website.

See below.

Other Health Related Books by the Author
- The Reluctant Bowel
- A Weighty Issue
- Sleep, Perchance to Dream
- **The Journey: EDS and chronic pain**
- The MND diet: using nutrition to slow down the progress of neurodegeneration

- A Necessary Sorrow
- Treat infection Naturally
- Successful Aging
- Taking another Road: Pain: its causes and what can be done about it.
- Osteoarthritis and Pain

- Multiple Sclerosis Tamed
- A Treatment Strategy for Migraine

These can be found here on the author's page
https://www.amazon.co.uk/-/e/B07BPQZ5CD

Gelatin from bone broth
Ingredients
Pork hocks or split pigs' feet (your butcher will do this for you).

Method
Cover with cold water and add choice of herbs. Simmer until very tender. Remove the hocks or pig's feet and allow to cool. This will begin to form a gel as it does so.

Oxtail soup

Ingredients

Two oxtail about 4 inches in length
One diced onion
One celery stalk
A little oil
A bay leaf
Some thyme
Some black peppercorns – about ten

One tablespoon of tomato puree
10 fluid ounces of red wine
One and a half pints of beef stock
A little cornflour to thicken

Method

Fry chunks of oxtail in the oil until browned then put aside on a plate.
Cook vegetables for 4-5 minutes. Add herbs, tomato Puree and peppercorns (you can replace the peppercorns with a little chilli, if desired.
Add the rest of the ingredients. Bring to the boil.
Once boiled, simmer for 3 hours.
Strain the cooking liquid. Take out the oxtail.
Leave in the refrigerator overnight once cooled.
The following day, take the fat off the cooled stock. Discard this. Add the chunks of oxtail. Heat the soup gently and mix some cornflour with a little cold water before adding to the soup to thicken it.

Serve with chunks of bread.

The stock, when you take it out of the refrigerator, will have a jelly like consistency. This is the gelatin that helps to keep connective tissue and gut healthy.

Printed in Great Britain
by Amazon